MAXIMIZING YOUR FERTILITY

Tips and Strategies for Conceiving a Baby

By

Dr. Keven Smith

TABLE OF CONTENTS

INTRODUCTION

Fertility is the ability to conceive and give birth to offspring. It is an important aspect of reproductive health, and it can be influenced by a variety of factors including age, lifestyle, and medical conditions.

There are several key concepts related to fertility that are important to understand:
The process of releasing an egg from the ovary is known as ovulation. It typically occurs around the middle of a woman's menstrual cycle, and it is necessary for pregnancy to occur.

Fertile window: The fertile window is the time during a woman's menstrual cycle when she is most likely to get pregnant. It usually occurs a few days before and after ovulation.
Male fertility: Male fertility refers to a man's ability to father a child. It can be affected by a variety of factors including age, lifestyle, and medical conditions.

Infertility: Infertility is defined as the inability to get pregnant after trying for one year (or six months if the woman is over 35). It can be caused by a variety of factors, including hormonal imbalances, structural problems with the reproductive system, and lifestyle factors.

It's important to note that fertility can vary widely from person to person, and there are many different factors that can influence it. It is always a good idea to speak with a healthcare provider if you have any questions or concerns about your fertility.

CHAPTER ONE: DEFINITION OF FERTILITY

Fertility is the ability to produce offspring. In humans, fertility refers to the ability to conceive and give birth to a child. It can be measured by the number of successful pregnancies a person or couple is able to have over a given period of time. Factors that can affect fertility include age, hormonal imbalances, certain medical conditions, and lifestyle factors such as smoking, drug use, and unhealthy diet and exercise habits. In women, fertility is typically at its highest in the early 20s and begins to decline after the age of 35. In men, fertility tends to remain relatively stable until the age of 40, after which it may decline.

Factors that can affect fertility There are many factors that can affect fertility in both men and women. Here are some of the most common:

1. Age: Fertility tends to decline with age, particularly for women over the age of 35.

2. Weight: Being underweight or overweight can affect fertility, as can dramatic weight changes.

3. Lifestyle factors: Alcohol consumption, smoking, and drug use can all negatively impact fertility.

4. Medical conditions: Certain medical conditions, such as polycystic ovary syndrome (PCOS) and endometriosis, can make it more difficult for a woman to get pregnant. For men, conditions such as low sperm count or varicoceles (enlarged veins in the scrotum) can affect fertility.

5. Hormonal imbalances: Hormonal imbalances can affect fertility in both men and women. For example, low testosterone levels in men or irregular periods in women may indicate a hormonal imbalance.

6.STIs: Some sexually transmitted infections (STIs) can cause inflammation of the reproductive organs and lead to fertility problems.

7. Stress: High levels of stress can affect fertility by disrupting the production of hormones that are necessary for reproduction.

8. Environmental factors: Exposure to certain toxins or chemicals, such as pesticides and lead, can affect fertility.

9. Genetics: Inherited conditions, such as chromosomal abnormalities, can affect fertility.

It's important to note that these are just some of the many factors that can affect fertility. If you are having trouble getting pregnant, it's a good idea to speak with a healthcare provider to determine the cause and discuss treatment options.

Understanding fertility in men and women Fertility in men and women refers to the ability to produce offspring. In men, fertility involves the production of healthy sperm, which are the male reproductive cells that are responsible for fertilizing a woman's egg during sexual reproduction. In women, fertility involves the production of healthy eggs, which are the female reproductive cells that are capable of being fertilized by a man's sperm.

There are several factors that can affect fertility in both men and women, including age, lifestyle factors such as diet and exercise, and certain medical conditions. For example, as men and women age, their fertility tends to decline. In women, fertility is highest in the 20s and early 30s and begins to decline gradually after the age of 35. In men, fertility begins to decline after the age of 40, but the decline is typically more gradual than in women.

Lifestyle factors can also affect fertility. For example, smoking, alcohol consumption, and drug use can all negatively impact fertility. Additionally, certain medical conditions can affect fertility, such as sexually transmitted infections, hormonal imbalances, and chronic health conditions such as diabetes.

If you are trying to conceive, it is important to be aware of any factors that may affect your fertility and to discuss them with your healthcare provider. There are also various medical treatments that can help improve fertility, such as fertility medications and assisted reproductive technologies such as in vitro fertilization (IVF).

Factors that affect fertility: There are many factors that can affect fertility in both men and women. Some of the main factors that can affect fertility include:

Age: Fertility tends to decline with age, especially in women. Women are most fertile in their 20s and early 30s, and fertility begins to decline more rapidly after the age of 35. Men can also experience a decline in fertility as they get older, although it tends to happen later in life than it does for women.

Weight: Both underweight and overweight conditions might impact fertility. Being underweight can cause irregular periods or stop periods altogether, which can make it difficult to get pregnant. Being overweight can also cause fertility problems, as excess weight can cause hormonal imbalances that can affect ovulation.

Health conditions: Certain health conditions, such as polycystic ovary syndrome (PCOS), endometriosis, and uterine fibroids, can affect fertility. In men, health conditions such as low sperm count, abnormal sperm shape or motility, and erectile dysfunction can also affect fertility.
Lifestyle factors: A number of lifestyle factors can affect fertility, including smoking, alcohol consumption, drug use, and stress. All of these can have a negative impact on reproductive health.

Medications: Some medications can affect fertility, either by reducing sperm count or disrupting ovulation. If you are trying to get pregnant, it is important to talk to your doctor about any medications you are taking and whether they might affect your fertility.
Age and fertility Fertility tends to decrease with age in both men and women. In women, fertility starts to

decline in their early 20s and decreases more rapidly after age 35. By age 40, a woman's fertility has significantly decreased, and it continues to decline as she gets older.

In men, fertility also decreases with age, but the decline is not as steep as it is in women. While male fertility remains relatively high until age 50 or so, it starts to decline gradually after age 40.

CHAPTER TWO: THERE ARE SEVERAL FACTORS THAT CONTRIBUTE TO THE DECLINE IN FERTILITY WITH AGE, INCLUDING:

Decreased egg quality and quantity in women
Decreased sperm quality and quantity in men
Changes in the reproductive system that can affect fertility
If you are trying to get pregnant and are concerned about your fertility, it is a good idea to talk to a healthcare provider. They can help you understand your fertility potential and discuss options for conceiving, such as fertility treatments or assisted reproductive technologies.

Health and fertility There are many factors that can affect health and fertility. Here are some things to think about: Nutrition Eating a healthy, balanced diet can support overall health and fertility. This includes getting enough of key nutrients like folic acid, iron, and zinc.

Exercise: Staying active through regular exercise can help maintain a healthy weight, which can support fertility. However, extreme or intense exercise may have negative effects on fertility.

Sleep: Adequate sleep is important for overall health, including fertility.

Stress: Chronic stress can have negative effects on fertility, so finding ways to manage stress, such as through relaxation techniques or therapy, may be helpful.

Weight: Being overweight or underweight can affect fertility. It's important to maintain a healthy weight for your height and body type.

Smoking and alcohol: Smoking and excessive alcohol consumption can have negative effects on fertility.

Age: Fertility naturally declines with age, and this can be a factor for both men and women.

If you're concerned about your fertility or want to learn more about how to optimize your health and fertility, it's a good idea to talk to a healthcare provider. They can provide personalized recommendations based on your specific needs and circumstances.

Lifestyle and fertility Lifestyle can have a significant impact on fertility. Here are some specific ways that lifestyle can affect fertility:

Weight: Being overweight or underweight can affect fertility. Being significantly overweight or obese can lead to hormonal imbalances that can affect ovulation and fertility while being underweight can lead to irregular periods or missed periods, which can also affect fertility.

Exercise: Moderate exercise is generally considered to be beneficial for fertility, but excessive or intense exercise can have the opposite effect. Overly strenuous exercise can lead to menstrual dysfunction and fertility problems.

Diet: A healthy diet is important for fertility. Some specific things to consider include getting enough protein, eating a variety of fruits and vegetables, and avoiding processed and sugary foods.

Stress: High levels of stress can affect fertility by altering hormone levels and disrupting menstrual cycles.

Alcohol and tobacco use: Excessive alcohol consumption and tobacco use can both negatively impact fertility.

Sleep: Getting enough sleep is important for overall health, including fertility.
It's worth noting that fertility can be affected by many factors, and lifestyle is just one of them. If you're concerned about your fertility, it's a good idea to speak with a healthcare provider for personalized advice and guidance.
Medical conditions and fertility There are many medical conditions that can affect fertility. Some common conditions that may impact fertility include:

Polycystic ovary syndrome (PCOS): This is a hormonal disorder that can cause irregular periods and make it difficult for a woman to ovulate.
Endometriosis: This is a condition in which tissue that normally lines the uterus grows outside of the uterus, causing pain and often leading to fertility problems.

Ovarian cysts: These are fluid-filled sacs that can develop on the ovaries and may interfere with ovulation.
Uterine fibroids: These are non-cancerous growths that can develop in the uterus and can cause infertility by

blocking the passage of eggs from the ovaries to the uterus.

Pelvic inflammatory disease (PID): This is an infection of the reproductive organs that can cause scarring and damage to the fallopian tubes, making it difficult for eggs to travel from the ovaries to the uterus.

Male factor infertility: This can be caused by various factors, including low sperm count, poor sperm quality, or other problems with the reproductive system.

It's important to note that many of these conditions can be treated, and fertility can often be restored with the help of medical intervention or assisted reproductive technologies. If you are experiencing fertility problems, it's a good idea to speak with a healthcare provider or a fertility specialist to discuss your options.

Medications and fertility There are several medications that can affect fertility in both men and women. It is important to discuss with a healthcare provider how any medication you are taking may impact your fertility.

In women, certain medications can disrupt the menstrual cycle and decrease the production of eggs, which can make it more difficult to get pregnant. These medications may include:

Birth control pills: These can alter the levels of hormones in the body, which can affect fertility.

Chemotherapy: Some chemotherapy drugs can damage the eggs or impair their production, which can lead to fertility problems.

Antidepressants: Some antidepressant medications can affect the levels of certain hormones in the body, which can affect fertility.

Opioids: Opioids, such as morphine and codeine, can affect fertility by altering the menstrual cycle and decreasing the production of eggs.

In men, certain medications can affect fertility by decreasing the production of sperm or impairing its movement. These medications may include:

Antidepressants: Some antidepressants can affect the production of sperm or its movement, which can affect fertility.

Opioids: Opioids can affect the production of testosterone, which is important for the production of sperm.

Chemotherapy: Some chemotherapy drugs can damage the cells that produce sperm, which can lead to fertility problems.

It is important to discuss with a healthcare provider any concerns you have about the potential impact of medications on your fertility. They can help you understand the potential risks and benefits of different treatment options and help you make an informed decision about your healthcare.

Fertility testing and evaluation: Fertility testing and evaluation is a process that helps people understand their fertility and identify potential fertility issues. It can be done for both men and women and may involve a combination of physical exams, blood tests, and other diagnostic procedures.

CHAPTER THREE: THERE ARE SEVERAL TYPES OF FERTILITY TESTS THAT CAN BE DONE:

Ovarian reserve testing: This involves testing the quality and quantity of a woman's eggs. It can be done with blood tests (such as follicle-stimulating hormone [FSH] and anti mullerian hormone [AMH] tests) and ultrasound.
Semen analysis: This involves evaluating the quality of a man's sperm, including the number, shape, and movement of the sperm.

Hormone testing: Hormone imbalances can affect fertility. Blood tests can check levels of hormones such as FSH, luteinizing hormone (LH), and testosterone.

Hysterosalpingography (HSG): This is an X-ray procedure that looks at the inside of the uterus and fallopian tubes to check for blockages or abnormalities.

Laparoscopy: This is a surgical procedure that allows a doctor to see inside the pelvis and look for problems such as scar tissue, endometriosis, or uterine abnormalities.

It's important to talk to a healthcare provider about which fertility tests are appropriate for you. Fertility testing and evaluation can help identify any potential issues that may be causing difficulties in conceiving and can guide treatment decisions.

Fertility testing for men: Fertility testing for men can help determine if there are any issues that may be contributing to fertility problems or infertility. There are several tests that can be used to evaluate a man's fertility, including:

Semen analysis: This is the most common fertility test for men. It involves collecting a semen sample and evaluating the number, shape, and movement of the sperm.

Hormonal testing: Hormone imbalances can affect fertility, so a blood test may be done to measure levels of hormones such as testosterone, follicle-stimulating hormone (FSH), and luteinizing hormone (LH).

Genetic testing: Some men may have genetic abnormalities that can affect fertility. Genetic testing can identify these abnormalities and help guide treatment.

Physical examination and medical history: A physical examination and review of medical history can help identify any physical issues that may be contributing to fertility problems, such as varicoceles or sexually transmitted infections.

It's important to note that fertility testing for men is usually done in conjunction with fertility testing for women, as fertility issues can be caused by factors in both partners. If fertility problems are identified, a reproductive endocrinologist or fertility specialist can work with the couple to determine the best course of treatment.

Fertility testing for women: Fertility testing for women typically involves several different types of tests, which may be performed individually or in combination. These tests can help to identify any issues that may be affecting a woman's fertility and guide treatment options. Some common fertility tests for women include:

Ovulation testing: This involves checking for signs of ovulation, such as changes in basal body temperature or the presence of certain hormones in the urine. Ovulation testing can help to determine whether a woman is ovulating regularly, which is important for fertility.

Hormone testing: Hormone testing can help to identify any hormonal imbalances that may be affecting fertility. This may include testing for levels of follicle-stimulating hormone (FSH), luteinizing hormone (LH), and estrogen.

Pelvic ultrasound: A pelvic ultrasound is a non-invasive test that uses sound waves to create an image of the pelvic organs. This test can help to identify any structural abnormalities in the uterus or ovaries that may be causing fertility issues.

Hysterosalpingography (HSG): This test involves injecting a special dye into the uterus and then taking an X-ray to see if the dye passes through the fallopian tubes. This test can help to identify any blockages or abnormalities in the fallopian tubes, which can affect fertility.

Laparoscopy: A laparoscopy is a surgical procedure in which a small camera is inserted through a small incision in the abdomen to examine the pelvic organs. This test can help to identify any structural abnormalities or other issues that may be affecting fertility.

It's important to note that fertility testing is just one step in the process of diagnosing and treating fertility issues. Other factors, such as age, overall health, and lifestyle, can also play a role in fertility. If you're concerned about your fertility, it's a good idea to speak with a healthcare provider or fertility specialist for personalized advice and treatment options.

Understanding fertility test results There are several types of fertility tests that can be used to evaluate a person's ability to conceive. The results of these tests can provide important information about a person's fertility and help identify any potential fertility issues.

Some common fertility tests for men include semen analysis, which evaluates the quality and quantity of sperm, and hormone testing, which measures levels of hormones such as testosterone and follicle-stimulating hormone (FSH).

Fertility tests for women may include hormone testing to evaluate levels of hormones such as estrogen, progesterone, and FSH, as well as testing for the presence of ovulatory disorders. Other tests for women may include imaging tests, such as an ultrasound, to evaluate the uterus and fallopian tubes, or a laparoscopy, which is a surgical procedure used to examine the reproductive organs.

It's important to interpret fertility test results in the context of a person's medical history and other factors and to discuss the results with a healthcare provider. A healthcare provider can help explain the test results and provide guidance on the next steps, which may include lifestyle changes, medication, or other treatments.

Fertility treatments: Fertility treatments are medical procedures or medications used to help people become pregnant. There are many different fertility treatments available, and the right one for you will depend on your individual circumstances. Some common fertility treatments include:

Ovulation induction: This involves taking medications to stimulate the ovaries to produce eggs.

Intrauterine insemination (IUI): This involves placing sperm directly into the uterus around the time of ovulation to increase the chances of fertilization.

In vitro fertilization (IVF): This involves fertilizing an egg with sperm in a laboratory dish and then transferring the resulting embryo to the uterus.

Intracytoplasmic sperm injection (ICSI): This is a type of IVF in which a single sperm is injected directly into an egg. It is often used when the man has a low sperm count or poor sperm quality.

Surrogacy: This involves using another woman to carry a pregnancy to term for someone who is unable to carry a pregnancy themselves.

It's important to talk to a fertility specialist or reproductive endocrinologist to determine the best fertility treatment plan for you. They can help you understand the potential risks and benefits of different treatment options and help you make an informed decision.

Medications to boost fertility There are several medications that can be used to boost fertility in both men and women. Here are a few examples:

Clomiphene citrate: This is a medication that is commonly used to treat infertility in women. It works by stimulating the production of hormones that regulate ovulation.

Gonadotropins: These medications contain hormones that stimulate the production of eggs in the ovaries. They are often used in combination with other fertility treatments, such as in vitro fertilization (IVF).

Metformin: This medication is often used to treat type 2 diabetes, but it can also be used to treat polycystic ovary syndrome (PCOS), a common cause of infertility in women.

Letrozole: This medication is used to treat breast cancer, but it can also be used off-label to stimulate ovulation in women with fertility problems.

Tamoxifen: Like letrozole, tamoxifen is a medication that is used to treat breast cancer, but it can also be used off-label to stimulate ovulation in women with fertility problems.

It's important to note that fertility medications can have side effects and may not be suitable for everyone. It's always best to discuss your treatment options with a fertility specialist or healthcare provider.

Assisted reproductive technologies (ART) Assisted reproductive technologies (ART) refer to a group of medical procedures used to help couples or individuals who are unable to conceive a child naturally to have a baby. ART includes a range of treatments such as in vitro fertilization (IVF), gamete intrafallopian transfer (GIFT), and intracytoplasmic sperm injection (ICSI).

IVF is a process in which eggs are fertilized with sperm outside of the body, in a laboratory dish. The fertilized eggs, or embryos, are then transferred back into the woman's uterus to implant and grow.

GIFT is a procedure in which eggs and sperm are placed together in the fallopian tubes, where fertilization occurs naturally.

ICSI involves injecting a single sperm into an egg in a laboratory dish to fertilize it. The resulting embryo is then transferred to the uterus.

These procedures can be effective in helping people who have fertility problems due to a variety of factors, such as blocked or damaged fallopian tubes, low sperm count, or problems with the uterus or ovaries. However, they are not always successful and may not be an option for everyone. It's important to discuss the potential risks and benefits with a medical professional before deciding whether to pursue ART.

Surgical procedures to improve fertility There are several surgical procedures that can be used to improve fertility in men and women. These procedures are typically used to correct physical abnormalities or to remove blockages that are preventing the egg and sperm from coming into contact.

In women, some common surgical procedures include:

Laparoscopy: This procedure involves making a small incision in the abdomen and inserting a laparoscope (a thin, lighted tube) to view the reproductive organs. The surgeon can then diagnose and treat any problems they see, such as endometriosis or scar tissue.

Hysteroscopy: This procedure involves inserting a thin, lighted tube through the cervix to view the inside of the uterus. The surgeon can then remove any growths or abnormalities they see, such as uterine fibroids or polyps.

Fallopian tube surgery: This procedure involves repairing or removing damaged fallopian tubes, which can be a cause of infertility.

In men, some common surgical procedures include:

Vasectomy reversal: This procedure involves reversing a vasectomy, which is a form of permanent birth control that involves cutting and sealing the vas deferens (the tubes that carry sperm from the testicles to the penis).

Varicocele repair: This procedure involves repairing damaged veins in the scrotum, which can cause fertility problems.

Testicular surgery: This procedure involves removing a blockage or repairing damaged tissue in the testicles, which can be a cause of infertility.

It's important to note that these are just a few examples of surgical procedures that may be used to improve fertility. The specific procedure recommended for a particular individual will depend on their unique circumstances and fertility problems.

Coping with fertility challenges: Dealing with fertility challenges can be emotionally and physically challenging. It is important to remember that you are not alone and that there are many resources available to help you cope. Here are a few things that may be helpful:

Seek support: Talk to your partner, family, friends, or a therapist about your feelings and concerns. It can be helpful to have someone to talk to who understands what you are going through.

Educate yourself: Learning more about fertility and the various treatment options can help you make informed decisions about your care.

Take care of yourself: Make sure to eat a healthy diet, get enough sleep, and exercise regularly to keep your body in good shape.

Consider alternative options: If you are struggling to get pregnant, you may want to consider alternative options such as adoption or surrogacy.

Seek professional help: If you are having difficulty coping with fertility challenges, consider seeking help from a mental health professional who can provide you with support and guidance.

Remember, it is important to take care of yourself and seek support when needed. There are many resources available to help you cope with fertility challenges, and you do not have to go through this difficult time alone.

Emotional support for fertility challenges I'm sorry to hear that you're facing fertility challenges. It's natural to feel a range of emotions when dealing with fertility issues, and it's important to remember that it's okay to feel overwhelmed, sad, angry, or frustrated.

CHAPTER FOUR: HERE ARE FEW TIPS THAT MAY HELP YOU COPE WITH YOUR EMOTIONS:

Find a support system: It can be helpful to talk to friends, family, or a therapist about your feelings. It's important to have people you can lean on and who will listen to you.

Practice self-care: Taking care of yourself can help you feel better emotionally and physically. This might include activities such as exercising, getting enough sleep, and eating well.

Seek out resources: There are many resources available to help you cope with fertility challenges. These may include support groups, therapy, and fertility clinics.

Be kind to yourself: It's important to remember that you are not alone in your fertility journey and that it's okay to have ups and downs. Try to be patient with yourself and practice self-compassion.

I hope these suggestions are helpful. Please don't hesitate to reach out if you have any questions or if you would like to talk more about your feelings.

Coping with fertility treatments Undergoing fertility treatment can be an emotionally and physically challenging experience. Here are a few tips that may help you cope with the process:

Find support: It can be helpful to talk to others who are going through similar experiences. This could be a support group, a therapist, or friends and family.

Take care of yourself: Make sure to prioritize self-care during this time. Eat a healthy diet, exercise regularly, and get enough rest. It may also be helpful to try stress-reducing activities such as meditation or yoga.

Communicate with your partner: It's important to keep lines of communication open with your partner throughout the fertility treatment process. Talk about your feelings and concerns, and make sure to support each other.

Set realistic expectations: It's natural to hope for the best, but it's important to be realistic about the chances of success with fertility treatment. It may help to have open and honest conversations with your healthcare provider about your options and the likelihood of success.

Seek help if you need it: If you're struggling to cope with the emotional aspects of fertility treatment, don't hesitate to seek help from a mental health professional. They can provide you with the support and guidance you need to get through this challenging time.

Alternative approaches to fertility may consider if they are having difficulty conceiving or wish to have children through non-traditional means. Some of these options include:

Adoption: Adoption is the process of legally becoming the parent of a child who is not biologically related to you. There are several types of adoption, including domestic adoption (within the same country) and international adoption (from another country).

Surrogacy: Surrogacy is a fertility treatment in which a woman carries and gives birth to a baby on behalf of another person or couple. There are two types of surrogacy: gestational surrogacy, in which the surrogate carries an embryo created using the intended parents' or donors' eggs and sperm, and traditional surrogacy, in which the surrogate's own egg is fertilized using the intended father's sperm.

Egg or sperm donation: Egg or sperm donation is a fertility treatment in which a woman donates her eggs or a man donates his sperm to be used in assisted reproduction, such as in vitro fertilization (IVF).

Co-parenting: Co-parenting is a non-romantic relationship in which two or more individuals agree to have and raise a child together. Co-parenting arrangements can be informal or legally recognized.

It is important to carefully consider the potential risks and benefits of these alternative approaches to fertility and to discuss them with a healthcare provider or mental health professional.

Maintaining good reproductive health: Maintaining good reproductive health involves taking care of your physical and emotional well-being, as well as adopting healthy behaviors to prevent reproductive health problems. The following advice can help you maintain good reproductive health:1.Practice safe sex: Using condoms or other forms of protection can help prevent sexually transmitted infections (STIs) and unintended pregnancies.

2. Get vaccinated: Some vaccines can protect against STIs, such as the human papillomavirus (HPV) vaccine.

3. Get regular check-ups: Regular check-ups with a healthcare provider can help identify and address any reproductive health concerns early on.

4. Eat a healthy diet: A balanced diet rich in fruits, vegetables, and other nutrients can support overall health and reproductive health.

5. Exercise regularly: Regular physical activity can help maintain a healthy weight and improve overall health.

6. Practice stress management: Chronic stress can affect reproductive health, so it's important to find ways to manage stress, such as through exercise, meditation, or talking to a therapist.

7. Avoid smoking and excessive alcohol consumption: These behaviors can negatively impact reproductive health.

8. Know your body: Pay attention to any changes or abnormalities in your reproductive system, and report any concerns to your healthcare provider.

By following these tips, you can help maintain good reproductive health and reduce your risk of

Tips for maintaining good reproductive health
Preconception care: Preconception care is a type of healthcare that focuses on preparing for pregnancy before it occurs. It involves taking steps to improve your overall health and fertility, as well as reducing any potential risks to your future pregnancy.

Some steps you can take to prepare for pregnancy include:
Visit your healthcare provider: It's a good idea to make an appointment with your healthcare provider before trying to get pregnant. Your provider can help you assess your current health, discuss any potential risks or concerns, and recommend any necessary lifestyle changes or medical interventions.

Make healthy lifestyle choices: Adopting a healthy lifestyle is important for both your overall health and the health of your future baby. This includes eating a well-balanced diet, getting regular physical activity, avoiding smoking and excessive alcohol consumption, and managing stress.

Take folic acid: Folic acid is a B vitamin that is important for the development of the neural tube, which becomes the brain and spinal cord. It is recommended that women who are planning to become pregnant take a daily supplement of at least 400 micrograms of folic acid.

Manage chronic conditions: If you have any chronic health conditions, such as diabetes or epilepsy, it's important to manage these conditions carefully before and during pregnancy. Your healthcare provider can help you develop a plan to optimize your health and minimize any potential risks to your pregnancy.

Preconception care is important because it can help improve your chances of having a healthy pregnancy and a healthy baby. If you are thinking about becoming pregnant, it's a good idea to talk to your healthcare provider about your plans and any steps you can take to prepare for pregnancy.

CONCLUSION:

There are many different fertility challenges that individuals and couples may face. These can be caused by a variety of factors, including age, health conditions, lifestyle factors, and genetics. It is important for individuals and couples who are experiencing fertility challenges to seek medical advice and support to help them understand the causes of their fertility issues and explore potential treatment options. Some common fertility challenges include:

Ovulatory disorders: These are problems with the production and release of eggs from the ovaries.

Male factor infertility: This refers to problems with the production or delivery of sperm.

Endometriosis: This is a condition in which tissue that normally lines the uterus grows outside of the uterus, which can cause problems with fertility.

Polycystic ovary syndrome (PCOS): This is a hormonal disorder that can cause irregular periods and make it difficult to get pregnant.

Uterine or cervical abnormalities: These include problems with the shape or structure of the uterus or cervix, which can affect fertility.

Age-related fertility decline: Fertility naturally declines with age, and this can be a significant challenge for older individuals or couples trying to get pregnant.

There are many treatment options available for fertility challenges, including medication, surgery, and assisted reproductive technologies such as in vitro fertilization (IVF). The best course of action will depend on the specific fertility challenge being faced and the individual's personal circumstances.

Summary of key points:
 Here are some key points to consider when it comes to fertility challenges:

Fertility challenges can be caused by a variety of factors, including age, health conditions, lifestyle factors, and genetics.

Common fertility challenges include ovulatory disorders, male factor infertility, endometriosis, polycystic ovary syndrome (PCOS), uterine or cervical abnormalities, and age-related fertility decline.

It is important for individuals and couples experiencing fertility challenges to seek medical advice and support to understand the causes of their fertility issues and explore treatment options.

There are many treatment options available for fertility challenges, including medication, surgery, and assisted reproductive technologies such as in vitro fertilization (IVF).

The best course of action will depend on the specific fertility challenge being faced and the individual's personal circumstances.
Next steps for those seeking to improve their fertility: There are several steps that individuals seeking to improve their fertility can take:

Keep a healthy weight: Obesity and being underweight can both impact fertility. It is important to maintain a healthy weight through a balanced diet and regular exercise.
Quit smoking and avoid alcohol: Smoking and heavy alcohol consumption can negatively impact fertility. Quitting smoking and reducing alcohol intake may improve fertility.

Reduce stress: High levels of stress can affect fertility. Techniques such as meditation, yoga, and exercise can help reduce stress.

Get enough sleep: Getting enough sleep is important for overall health and can also impact fertility.
Consider fertility treatments: If you have been trying to get pregnant for an extended period of time without success, you may want to consider fertility treatments such as in vitro fertilization (IVF).

Seek medical advice: If you are having difficulty getting pregnant, it is important to speak with a healthcare provider to determine the cause and discuss possible treatment options.

It is also important to remember that fertility can be affected by a variety of factors, including age, medical conditions, and lifestyle choices. It is always a good idea to speak with a healthcare provider to determine the best course of action for improving fertility.